EAT TO LOWER BLOOD PRESSURE

Whole Foods That Helped Me Conquer Hypertension and Discontinue the Use of Medication in My 50s.

By
DR. NICOLINE AMBE

EAT TO LOWER BLOOD PRESSURE

Whole Foods That Helped Me Conquer Hypertension and Discontinue the Use of Medication in My 50s.

Copyright © 2024 by Nicoline Ambe

All rights reserved: No part of this publication may be reproduced, stored in a retrieval system, or transmitted in any form or by any means, electronic, mechanical, photocopying, recording, scanning, or otherwise, except as permitted by Sections 107 or 108 of the 1976 United States Copyright Act, without either the prior written permission of the copyright holder.

Printed in the United States of America

DEDICATION

This book is dedicated to everyone struggling with high blood pressure. May you find your healing.

ACKNOWLEDGEMENTS

Thank you to my daughters for their unconditional love and support. Thank God for leading me to the answers to lower my high blood pressure and avoid heart disease.

TABLE OF CONTENTS

DISCLAIMER	1
BACKGROUND	3
CHAPTER 1: The Dangers of High Blood Pressure	7
CHAPTER 2: Eat to Lower Blood Pressure	15
CHAPTER 3: Vegetables	23
CHAPTER 4: Fruits	31
CHAPTER 5: Healthy Fats	37
CHAPTER 6: Proteins	41
CHAPTER 7: Carbohydrates	45
CHAPTER 8: Spices and Herbs	49
CHAPTER 9: Beverages	53
CHAPTER 10: Supplement Your Diet	59
CONCLUSION: Toxin-free food	65
2 MONTHS BLOOD PRESSURE ROUTINE	73
LAST WORDS	99
ABOUT THE AUTHOR	101

DISCLAIMER

I am not a medical doctor. I am not giving you clinical advice. This book is not a scientific study – it doesn't have any scientific facts, research, citations, or quotations. Please consult your physician and do your research before applying anything you read in this book. Consider what works for your body and create a healthy plan for your everyday life that works for you. I am simply sharing ideas that have helped me lower and normalize my blood pressure, get off medication, improve my heart health, and win the battle against high blood pressure. I'm not trying to prove anything to anyone. I'm just telling my story.

I used to be stricken by many health issues, but I bounced back. I no longer have high blood pressure, palpitations, gut issues, headaches, tinnitus, fatigue, dental problems, back pain, nerve pain, blurry vision, or debilitating hormonal dysfunctions. I am no longer on any prescription medication. I feel better than I have ever felt in years. Changing my diet, specifically by adding more whole foods to my meal plan, worked well for me. I am not saying this has to be your plan. This is my plan, and it has worked miracles for me.

DISCLAIMER

Getting older is never a justification for sickness or an excuse to suffer from metabolic disorders like high blood pressure. We have choices – we can choose to change our health conditions with the proper diet and lifestyle modification. We are in complete control of our health. This is my belief. If you see yourself in me, I invite you to accompany me on this journey to normal blood pressure and excellent heart health. It is a learning process. It is also a complex process that requires discipline, consistency, and tenacity. Be ready to try new things, feel frustrated, fail, and make mistakes until you discover what works best for your body. Are you ready? Let's blossom…

BACKGROUND

In 2016, at forty-eight years of age, I checked in to Urgent Care with a blood pressure of 167/101. The doctor put me on medication to control it. The treatment consisted of 10 mg of Lisinopril. I was on that medication for four years. In March 2020, I decided to stop taking the medication because I did not like the side effects – coughing and frequent urination. It also felt like something foreign was living in my body. I was never at ease!

During the time I was on the medication, and shortly after stopping it, I developed strange issues with my health that included the following:

- Gut issues
- High blood sugar
- Tinnitus (ringing in the head)
- Tooth and gum problems
- Blurry vision
- Pressure on my left eye and weakening of the eye
- Nerve pain in my legs
- Back pain

BACKGROUND

- Arthritis
- Belly fat
- Fatigue
- Painful joints
- Forgetfulness

Dealing with all of the above, including the side effects of the medication, took a toll on my body. I wasn't sure if these issues caused the high blood pressure or if high blood pressure was the cause and the role of the medication in all of this. I could not figure out the interconnection. I felt horrible but had no answers, yet I didn't want to keep taking medication. Honestly, I knew that if I kept going without a clear plan for taking charge of my health, something terrible would happen within five years.

In 2020, I drew a line in the sand. Every day, I was sick and tired of feeling sick and tired. I began my healing journey by reading books and researching to find answers to my health woes, which I later learned were triggered by uncontrolled high blood pressure. I attended seminars, followed holistic physicians on social media, and purchased several health books from doctors and wellness practitioners. Much of the information I gathered were general tips on eating whole foods and lifestyle modification. I was looking for something more specific to lower my blood pressure - a clear plan - not generic information I could not implement. I did not find information on a complete program to follow. Like most people, I felt lost in a sea of information and still didn't have the answer to lower my blood pressure and get off medication. I needed to know more.

In August 2021, I enrolled in a health coaching school (HCI) to deepen my knowledge and understanding of health, wellness, and healing. While in health coaching school, I focused on heart disease, high blood pressure, high cholesterol, and what to eat for a healthy heart. The more I researched and dug into these areas, the closer I got to the answer.

I've come full circle and have been off medication since 2020. Having mastery over my body, I monitor my blood pressure at home twice daily. On average, it is 115/77. I know what to eat or drink to lower it when it's rising during the day. I know how it feels when it is high and what to do about it. I feel better than I did at twenty-four. My mission is to help adults over 50 who are struggling with chronic metabolic syndrome to get in the best shape of their lives and lower their blood pressure, blood sugar, and cholesterol so they can avoid chronic health conditions, enjoy renewed vitality, and blossom at any age.

This book gives you the plan – my plan. It doesn't just give you general information or leave you wondering how to pair foods and what foods to eat; it provides a sample eating routine you can follow daily and make your own. Eating to lower blood pressure is not the usual way to eat. It takes discipline and a strong desire to change to follow an eating plan to lower your blood pressure. The

BACKGROUND

book also discusses effective lifestyle habits you can immediately implement to strengthen your heart.

As you embark on this journey to wellness and healing from high blood pressure, think of the things that motivate you - why you wake up every morning - your passion, purpose, family, goals, mental health, retirement years, etc. Let these things inspire you to give your best to restore your health. So many people fall off the wagon of good health due to a lack of motivation, vision for their future, and old habits that keep them trapped. I know this is not you.

There's no doubt you have been through hard struggles in your life. Eating and making lifestyle changes to lower your blood pressure isn't above or beneath you. You can do hard things. You can do this! Optimizing your heart health is personal to me. I've walked a mile in your shoes and know where it hurts. I have learned how to make a comeback from debilitating health issues to enjoying a healthy, purposeful, vibrant, and medication-free life. Know that you're not alone on this journey. I'm here to support you in all the ways I can. As you begin your new lifestyle habits, please use your physician as a resource and notify them of your decisions and progress.

Now, let's look at the dangers of high blood pressure...

CHAPTER 1

The Dangers of High Blood Pressure

High blood pressure is a serious condition that increases the risk of coronary heart disease, stroke, kidney failure, heart attack, and other health problems. Blood pressure is the force of blood pushing against arterial walls while the heart pumps out blood. A strong force over an extended period is called high blood pressure. Left untreated, high blood pressure damages and scars the arteries.

Blood flows easily through healthy arteries when they are smooth and flexible. When the heart beats, it forces blood through the arteries to the rest of the body and its organs. The more forceful the blood pumps are, the more the arteries stretch and allow blood to flow easily. When blood pressure is too high, or if blood flow is too forceful, this flexible tissue that makes up the arterial walls will be stretched beyond a healthy limit. Over time, high blood pressure can damage the blood vessel walls, causing them to malfunction.

Fats in the blood (from the food we eat) can collect in these damaged arteries, clogging them up and leading to what is known as atherosclerosis. Atherosclerosis is the thickening or hardening of the arteries caused by a buildup of plaque in the inner lining of an artery. This thickening and hardening will cause the arteries to become narrow and stiff. Eventually, the arteries become too narrow for enough blood to flow around the body and organs. The narrowing and blocking of the arteries can cause cardiovascular diseases, which include coronary artery disease (CAD).

CAD occurs when the arteries leading to the heart are narrowed or blocked, causing chest pain or heart attacks. This narrowing can also cause peripheral artery disease (PAD) when too little blood reaches the legs and feet, making walking painful. Another possible outcome of narrow arteries is a stroke, where an artery to the brain is blocked or bursts. Another serious condition that can occur with atherosclerosis is the enlarging or weakening of the heart. This can lead to heart failure, a condition in which the heart cannot pump enough blood throughout the body.

Atherosclerosis can also cause the narrowing of blood vessels in the kidneys (which may cause kidney failure), bursting or bleeding of blood vessels in the eyes (possibly leading to blindness or vision changes), and so on. These are serious health conditions. Maintaining normal blood pressure or working to lower high blood pressure can significantly reduce your risk of developing more severe health issues.

EAT TO LOWER BLOOD PRESSURE

By making healthy changes to your lifestyle, you can improve the health of your heart. The whole foods in this book are rich in vitamins, minerals, and antioxidants that relax and dilate the arteries for better blood flow and mitigate the causes of high blood pressure. Creating healthy daily habits can also help you enjoy a stress-free life and a healthy heart.

Know Your Numbers

About 47% of adults in the United States have high blood pressure, and 20% do not know they have the condition. High blood pressure has no apparent symptoms; it can damage the heart, blood vessels, kidneys, and other body parts for years without any obvious signs. As a result, knowing your blood pressure numbers is important, despite how you feel physically. You should, therefore, take the necessary steps to lower your blood pressure if it's too high. People often learn that they have high blood pressure only after they experience a heart attack or stroke or develop heart disease. Having your blood pressure checked regularly and knowing your numbers is crucial in preventing damage or serious health problems.

The numbers that determine blood pressure readings are systolic pressure (when the heart is pumping blood) and diastolic pressure (when the heart is resting between beats). Your blood pressure will often be written and stated as systolic over diastolic. A normal reading should be 120/80 mmHg.

THE DANGERS OF HIGH BLOOD PRESSURE

The risk factors of high blood pressure include the following:

- Obesity
- Race and ethnicity
- Unhealthy lifestyle habits
- Eating too much sodium in salty foods or drinks
- Drinking excess alcohol
- Insufficient potassium intake
- Insufficient magnesium intake
- Not enough exercise or physical activity
- Smoking
- A history of high blood pressure in the family
- Long periods of stress

When I had high blood pressure, I had difficulty knowing what to eat, in what combination, and at what time of day. Discovering these top blood pressure-fighting foods has been a miracle. However, whole foods are not the only way to lower blood pressure.

Below are important lifestyle changes to lower blood pressure:

- Eating a healthy diet
- Getting enough exercise
- Managing and learning to deal with stress.
- Ensuring quality sleep
- Effective Supplementation
- Maintaining a healthy body weight
- Quit smoking and avoid excessive alcohol.

EAT TO LOWER BLOOD PRESSURE

A healthy eating plan rich in fish, poultry, nuts, nutrients, protein, and fiber, low in sodium, fat, and cholesterol, and fewer sweets, added sugars, and sugar-containing beverages is the best approach to diet modification that lowers blood pressure. This book will give you an overview of the foods I have found to be the most effective for reducing blood pressure and improving heart health. It comes down to improving the health of the arteries and making them supple and adequately dilated. The foods I recommend eating contain antioxidants to heal not just the heart but also the body to do the following:

- Prevent oxidative stress.
- Regulate arterial blood pressure.
- Protect cells from premature aging.
- Enhance your immune system.
- Regulate digestive tract functions.
- Improve your bone health.

I encourage you to eat this way 95% of the time. When you implement the ideas in this book, not only will you lower your blood pressure and avoid heart disease, stroke, and heart attack, but you will also become younger, trimmer, sexier, mentally sharper, and healthier every day.

Living With High Blood Pressure

A high blood pressure diagnosis means you must treat and control it for the rest of your life. Even if treatment and lifestyle modification successfully lower your blood pressure, you still have the condition. Lifestyle changes will become a permanent part of your life, and although treatment helps to control blood pressure, it is not a cure.

Stopping treatment or lifestyle modification will raise your blood pressure again, which increases your risk for other health problems. Working toward a healthy future means following your treatment plan closely to gain lifelong control of high blood pressure. Therefore, keeping track of your blood pressure is vital. Have your blood pressure checked by your doctor or check it yourself at home. If you check it yourself at home, keep a journal and write down your numbers and the date each time you check your blood pressure. I have a blood pressure logbook you can purchase at **www.nicolineambe.com/books.** It will help you keep your readings in one place.

Why Most People Don't Heal

Many people want to lower their blood pressure and improve their cholesterol profiles (two leading causes of heart disease), but several things get in their way. Knowing why most people don't lower their blood pressure and stay on blood pressure medication for the rest of their lives might motivate you to change your behaviors and not be like most people. Statistics show that 1 in 3 people struggle with high blood pressure.

Here are the main reasons why so many people have difficulty lowering their blood pressure:

Lack of Motivation

Most people know what to do, meaning they should eat fruits and vegetables, exercise, sleep, and manage their stress levels. However, knowing what to do doesn't mean they will do it. They are not motivated to do what they know. To them, certain foods are more appealing and enticing than whole foods, so they choose comfort foods over healing foods.

Old Habits and Beliefs

I have no doubt you have heard the phrase, *"old habits die hard?"* Many people grew up with a habit of eating certain kinds of foods. For them, breaking old habits from their past can be difficult.

Making Excuses

Many people like making excuses and justifying their eating patterns and behaviors. My husband once believed he would have low energy if he didn't eat sugar. After looking at his doctor's report showing his cholesterol was high and he was pre-diabetic with high blood pressure, that belief changed instantly. Excuses will only get you so far before reality sets in.

Time Scarcity

Life is fast and can be hectic at times. Many people have limited time to plan and prepare healthy meals or practice important lifestyle habits because they often rush to work or deal with family demands.

Money Management

Many people would rather spend their money on fast food than prepare healthy meals at home. They would rather put premium fuel in their cars and drive through food in their bodies. The heart deserves premium fuel, too. Eating for the heart is an investment.

Lack of Knowledge

Many people need help with knowing what to do - what to eat, how to combine foods, what time of day to eat certain foods, how much to eat, and which nutrients to include in their diet.

Can you identify with any of these reasons why people don't develop the right plan to help them resolve their blood pressure issues? If you fall into any of these scenarios, start developing new habits to lower and manage your blood pressure and improve your health.

CHAPTER 2

Eat to Lower Blood Pressure

The goal of eating isn't to assuage hunger by impulsively filling your belly with food; it is to maintain and sustain your health. In fact, unknown to most people who think that *"nutrition"* means "to eat," the classic definition is *"the process of providing or obtaining the food necessary for health and growth."*

Good nutrition is essential for several reasons:

1. It adds more nutrients to nourish your body and promotes healthy bodily functions.
2. Provides antioxidants to combat inflammation.
3. Lowers the risk of chronic disease.
4. Promotes a healthy body weight.
5. Encourages the flushing out of toxins.

Good nutrition also means eating a healthy, balanced diet, which is essential for maintaining good health. It also means eating a wide variety of foods in the right proportions and consuming the right amount of food and drink to achieve and maintain a healthy body weight. In other words, a healthy diet is essential for good health and nutrition. It protects against chronic diseases like heart disease, diabetes, and cancer. Overall, eating the right variety of foods and consuming less salt, sugar, saturated, and industrially produced trans-fats are critical for a healthy diet.

My purpose with this section of the book is to promote good nutrition as a way for you to do the following:

- Lower blood pressure
- Achieve superior health.
- Maintain effective weight control.
- Reverse and prevent disease.

While weight control is important, it is not our primary focus. Instead, it is a significant by-product of lowering blood pressure and maintaining superior *health*. I accept that excessive weight is a significant problem for most people, but I have good news for these people. By applying those principles that will lead you to excellent health, you will naturally achieve your ideal weight.

These guidelines are designed to make you a *'nutrition expert'* yourself. Only by becoming an expert yourself can you achieve long-term success. That is because you will have learned how to cultivate new and healthy behaviors that will allow you to take control of your health and destiny.

The Objective of Good Nutrition

Good and balanced nutrition aims to increase the nutrient density of your diet. Read that twice! Most people don't get enough vitamins and minerals in their daily diet, leading to food cravings and overeating. It also makes them more susceptible to those serious diseases that have reached epidemic proportions in our society. Ultimately, I hope you will be able to adjust your diet so that you can start to lose your psychological dependence on unhealthy foods. The encouraging news is that you will reset your taste preferences and hunger drive by replacing unhealthy foods with nutrient-dense foods. Those who are overweight will be amazed at how easily they can and will lose weight without exerting strenuous effort at '*dieting,*' as we popularly know it.

Practical Tips on Healthy Eating

Eight practical tips cover the fundamentals of healthy eating that will help you make healthier choices. Always remember that the key to a healthy diet is to eat the right number of calories for how active you are so that you balance the energy you *consume* with the energy you *use*. Let us look at it from simple logic. You will gain weight if you eat or drink more than your body needs. This is because the extra energy, or calories, that you don't use is stored as fat.

You will lose weight if you eat and drink less than your body needs. This is because whatever fat you have will be burned off as calories to compensate for the shortfall and provide you with the energy you need for your activities. The daily recommended calorie intake for men is 2,500 calories. For women, it is 2,000. Additionally, eating a wide range of foods would ensure a balanced diet and that your body receives all the nutrients it needs. The keywords here are *energy* and *nutrients*.

1. Eat More Unrefined Carbohydrates

To achieve healthier outcomes for energy, choose high-fiber or whole-grain varieties of carbohydrates such as whole-grain pasta, brown rice, quinoa, wholewheat oats, potatoes with their skins on, whole-grain bread, popcorn, and breakfast cereal, winter squash, sweet potatoes, pumpkin, corn, and peas. They contain more fiber than white or refined starchy carbohydrates and can help you feel full longer.

Attempt to include at least one healthy carb with each main meal. These quality carbohydrates provide fewer than half the calories that starchy, refined carbohydrates provide. Be careful with the fats you use or add in cooking these foods. It is the fats that increase the calorie content.

2. Eat Lots of Fruits and Vegetables.

You should eat at least five portions of varieties of fruit and vegetables each day. This might sound daunting, but it is easier than it sounds, as you will discover in our routines. Fruits and vegetables benefit blood pressure because they are rich in nutrients like potassium, fiber, antioxidants, and other vitamins. The nutrients in these foods protect blood vessels from damage, improve blood flow, and reduce inflammation, all of which contribute to keeping blood pressure within the healthy range.

3. Eat More Healthy Fats

Healthy fats play a crucial role in managing and lowering blood pressure. Unsaturated fats help reduce inflammation and improve arterial health by keeping the arteries supple and flexible. Examples of healthy fats include Omega-3 fatty acids found in fish, flaxseeds, chia seeds, and walnuts. Other healthy fats are those rich in monounsaturated fats in foods like olive oil, avocados, and certain nuts. Not only do these healthy fats improve the health of the arteries, but they also help with nutrient absorption, reduce LDL cholesterol that can lead to plaque buildup in arteries, and have anti-inflammatory properties.

4. Reduce Your Intake of Saturated Fats

You must pay attention to the *amount* and *type* of fat you're eating. There are *two* main types of fat: *saturated and unsaturated*. Eating saturated fats can increase the amount of cholesterol in your blood, which will increase your risk of heart disease. Men should consume at most 30 grams of saturated fat a day. On average, women should consume no more than 20 grams of saturated fat daily.

Saturated fats are often considered unhealthy for the heart because they can raise levels of bad cholesterol and increase the risk of heart disease and cardiovascular issues like stroke and heart attack. Saturated fats are also known to promote inflammation in the body, which increases blood pressure and can cause chronic damage to the blood vessels. Many animal products are culpable and have a detrimental effect on the arteries. Limit the intake of fatty cuts of meat and many processed foods like butter, hard cheese, cream, cakes, biscuits, lard, pies, and full-fat dairy products. Instead, focus on a heart-healthy diet that includes unsaturated fats, plenty of fruits and vegetables, whole grains, and lean protein.

5. Reduce Your Intake of Sugar

Regularly consuming foods and drinks that are high in sugar increases your risk of obesity because sugary foods and beverages are high in calories. Free sugars are sugars added to foods or drinks or found naturally in honey, syrups, soda, and candy. This is the type of sugar you should avoid rather than the sugar in fruit. Many packaged foods and drinks contain surprisingly high amounts of free sugar. Free sugars are found in many foods, such as sugary fizzy drinks, sugary breakfast cereals, cakes, biscuits, pastries and puddings, sweets and chocolate, and alcoholic beverages. Food labels can help you check how much sugar foods contain. More than 22.5 grams of total sugar per 100 grams means the food is high in sugar, while 5 grams or less per 100 grams implies the food is low in sugar. However, the more you can avoid sugar, the better for you in the long run.

6. Consume Less Sodium

Your salt intake should be significantly limited, especially in adults over 50. Excessive consumption of salt can lead to elevated sodium levels in the body. High sodium levels can cause the body to retain water, thus raising blood pressure. Chronic hypertension is a significant risk factor for various cardiovascular diseases, such as heart attacks and strokes. Therefore, an intake of less than 2,300 mg per day, equal to 1 teaspoon of table salt, is often recommended as a preventive measure to help maintain healthy blood pressure levels and overall heart health.

7. Drink Plenty of Water

Refuse to get thirsty. The only way you can do this is by drinking plenty of fluids. Six to eight glasses of water are the daily recommendation, in addition to the fluid you obtain from your food. All non-alcoholic drinks count, but water, lower-fat milk, and lower-sugar drinks are healthier choices. Avoid sugary soft and fizzy drinks, as they are high in calories. Your combined total of drinks from fruit juice, vegetable juice, and smoothies should not be more than 150 ml daily (if at all), which is a small glass. Remember to drink even more fluids during hot weather or while exercising. Our routines outline a list of beverages that are suitable for blood pressure.

8. Practice Intermittent Fasting

While intermittent fasting may not be suitable for everyone, it does have many health benefits. Several studies have shown that intermittent fasting can help with weight loss, improved insulin sensitivity, balanced hormonal levels, reduced inflammation, and improved heart health, all contributing to lower blood pressure.

The next chapter on vegetables will summarize each vegetable, of which you should eat at least one serving a day to lower blood pressure and combat chronic diseases. This is not an exhaustive list of foods considered the most important. Most of these vegetables are classified as superfoods, and knowing them will set you off to a good start to eating for your blood pressure.

CHAPTER 3

Vegetables

Vegetables are an essential part of lowering high blood pressure. They are rich in fiber, vitamins, and nutrients that unclog and dilate arteries for improved blood flow and circulation. However, not all vegetables are the same when dealing with high blood pressure. The best vegetables for blood pressure are rich in nitrates, which convert to nitric oxide to dilate the arteries. This chapter shares the best vegetables for high blood pressure.

CABBAGE

All varieties of cabbage – red and green - are high in vitamin C, B6, folate, fiber, potassium, and vitamins. Cabbage can also raise beta-carotene, lutein, and other levels of heart-protective antioxidants. It also helps lower something called "oxidized" LDL, which is linked to the hardening of arteries. And since it eases inflammation, it can help prevent heart disease.

TIP: *Add extra crunch to your salads, soups, wraps, or sandwiches by topping them off with thinly sliced cabbage. Pump up the veggies on your hamburgers by adding slow-cooked cabbage, lettuce, tomatoes, pickles, and mayonnaise made with olive oil.*

BROCCOLI

Broccoli is a good source of magnesium, calcium, and potassium, three blood pressure-regulating minerals. It is loaded with flavonoids, an antioxidant that helps to lower blood pressure by enhancing blood vessel function and increasing nitric oxide levels in the body. A nutrient-rich vegetable, broccoli, may enhance your health in various ways, such as reducing inflammation, improving blood sugar control, boosting immunity, and promoting heart health. However, remember that good health doesn't come from any single food.

TIP: *To get maximum nutrients, steam broccoli in a steamer and sprinkle it with fresh lemon juice.*

CAULIFLOWER

Cauliflower is a heart-friendly vegetable rich in fiber and sulforaphane - a plant compound. Acting as an antioxidant, sulforaphane reduces the inflammatory damage caused by oxidative stress. Chronic inflammation can lead to arterial plaque and heart disease.

TIP: *Cut up the head of cauliflower and toss in olive oil, garlic powder, fresh ground black pepper, and a touch of Dijon mustard—roast in the oven at 375 degrees for 20 minutes. Remove and toss again, sprinkle with grated Parmesan cheese, and bake for another 15 minutes.*

KALE

Kale is rich in potassium, nitrate, fiber, folate, and calcium. Kale is also high in vitamins A and C. Vitamin K is essential for heart health. After we eat kale, the nitrates from the plant turn into nitric oxide, which dilates blood vessels and opens the arteries to lower blood pressure.

TIP: In a blender, add the following ingredients:

- ¼ cup of plain Kefir
- ½ cup of organic strawberries
- 1 green banana (purchase green bananas and peel them – store in the freezer)
- A handful of baby kale
- ½ cup of unsweetened vanilla almond milk
- Cinnamon to taste
- 2 tablespoons of peanut butter
- Ice

Blend well and enjoy.

BEETROOT

Beetroot contains nitrate, calcium, and vitamin A. These nutrients help to control blood pressure by dilating the arteries and allowing

VEGETABLES

for improved blood flow. Both raw beet juice and cooked beets effectively lower blood pressure and decrease inflammation.

TIP: When you purchase cooked beets, bring them home, place them in an airtight container, and pour apple cider vinegar overall. Add sliced beets to your favorite salad.

CELERY

Celery contains a phytochemical called phthalides. As an extract, it causes the tissues of the artery walls to increase blood flow and reduce blood pressure. It also contains folate and vitamin K, which are required to form red blood cells.

TIP: Add celery to your favorite salad or fill the crevice with almond butter for a quick snack.

TOMATOES

Tomatoes are rich in lycopene, potassium, vitamins B and E, and other nutrients. Lycopene is an anti-aging antioxidant that may help lower LDL cholesterol and blood pressure and improve heart health.

TIP: Add tomatoes to your favorite salad, make homemade tomato sauce, and toss with your favorite whole-grain pasta.

CARROTS

Carrots are an excellent source of vitamins A and K, potassium and fiber, vitamin C, calcium, and iron. The nutrients in carrots can help relax blood vessels and reduce inflammation, which may help lower blood pressure.

TIP: Toss baby carrots in olive oil, garlic powder, and thyme—roast in the oven at 350 degrees F for at least 30 minutes. Toss and roast for another 5-10 minutes. Enjoy as a snack.

CHARD

Swiss chard is a powerful source of vitamins A and C. It is also rich in potassium and magnesium and has high levels of nitrates, which have been shown to lower blood pressure.

TIP: Chard can be steamed or sauteed, and it's great in soups, stews, casseroles, frittatas, and quiches. Young leaves can be eaten raw in salads. Chard always has green leaves, but the stalks can be a variety of colors.

SPINACH

Spinach is rich in lutein, iron, and vitamin K. It is also rich in fiber and packed with heart-healthy nutrients like potassium, folate, and magnesium — critical ingredients for lowering and maintaining blood pressure levels.

TIP: Toss fresh spinach in a large skillet with olive, freshly chopped garlic, and freshly ground black pepper.

BRUSSELS SPROUT

Brussels sprouts are rich in vitamins C, K, folate, calcium, iron, and potassium. They're also rich in alpha-linolenic acid, converted to omega-3s in your body. These nutrients help improve blood flow, lower blood pressure, and prevent heart disease.

TIP: *Cut Brussels Sprouts in half. Toss in a bowl with olive oil and 2 chopped garlic cloves. Roast in a 375-degree oven for 40 minutes.*

ONIONS

Onions are rich in flavonoids and antioxidants that lower inflammation. Onions are also rich in vitamins A and C and are a great prebiotic food that controls inflammation, reduces the risk of heart attack, and prevents heart disease.

TIP: Add onions to salads, omelets, and sauces for flavor and nutrition.

LEEKS

Leeks are rich in flavonoids, an antioxidant that may improve digestion, reduce inflammation, and fight heart disease. The nutrients found in leeks contain heart-healthy plant compounds and are also shown to lower blood pressure and the formation of blood clots.

TIP: Leeks partner well with chicken, ham, cheese, cream, garlic, and shallots. Complementary herbs and spices include chervil, parsley, sage, thyme, basil, lemon, and mustard. Leeks can be fried, braised, boiled in soups or stocks, roasted in an oven, and even caramelized like onions.

ARUGULA

Arugula is rich in calcium, potassium, magnesium, vitamins C, K, A, and folate. Arugula is a nitrate-rich plant rich in antioxidants that can protect against cell and artery damage. Nitrates convert to nitric oxide to dilate the arteries for improved blood flow and lower blood pressure.

TIP: Arugula offers a delicious peppery flavor to any salad. It tastes good on a pizza with pesto, grilled chicken, diced tomatoes, garlic, and mushrooms.

DANDELION GREENS

Dandelion greens can be eaten cooked or raw and are an excellent source of vitamins A, C, and K. They also contain vitamin E, folate, and nitrates. Traditionally, dandelion was used as a diuretic to increase the amount of urine and eliminate fluid from the body.

TIP: White beans such as Cannellini, Great Northern, and Navy work nicely with dandelion greens. You can add the greens to a white bean salad, stew, or even soup for that extra flavor and nutrition. Just a nice citrusy vinaigrette will do the trick to balance the bitterness of a raw dandelion green salad.

ARTICHOKES

Artichokes are loaded with nutrients that may reduce high blood pressure by increasing nitric oxide to support arterial function and dilation. Research showed that artichoke leaf juice helped regulate blood pressure for people with mild high blood pressure.

TIP: The jarred variety is usually sold as marinated artichoke hearts, which are super flavorful and ready to eat.

COLLARD GREENS

Collard greens contain potassium and magnesium, essential minerals to control blood pressure. It is nutrient-dense and low in calories. They're an excellent source of calcium, folate, and vitamins K, C, and A, as well as high in fiber and antioxidants.

TIP: Like kale, collard greens are tough and fibrous, so cooking them until tender is necessary. You can cook the whole leaf and use it as a wrap for chicken salad.

BEET GREENS

Beet greens are a powerful source of vitamin K, vitamin A (in the form of carotenoids), vitamin C, copper, potassium, manganese, vitamin B2, and magnesium. Beet greens contain plenty of nitrates, which help lower blood pressure and improve oxygen levels.

TIP: Pair it with your favorite protein, pasta recipe, or soup, or serve it as part of a holiday dinner alongside classic dishes like sweet potato casserole, green bean casserole, mashed potatoes, and, of course, roasted beets.

As you can see, vegetables serve plenty of nutrients and can be easily added to your favorite foods and recipes.

In the next chapter, we will look at the endless health benefits of fruits...

CHAPTER 4

Fruits

Research suggests that eating fruit may lower the risk of cardiovascular diseases through its blood pressure-lowering effects. Eating the right fruit is extremely important for lowering blood pressure. Some fruits are higher in potassium than others, and these are the fruits that help to lower blood pressure and reduce the risk of heart disease.

BERRIES

Berries - blueberries, raspberries, blackberries, strawberries - are some of the healthiest fruits you can eat. They're low in calories and high in fiber, vitamin C, and antioxidants. Many berries have been associated with being beneficial for heart health. These include lowering blood pressure and reducing oxidative stress.

TIP: For a quick breakfast, berries are excellent to add to plain Greek yogurt with oats, grapes, and nuts.

BANANA

Bananas contain fiber, potassium, folate, and antioxidants like vitamin C. It protects the heart, strengthens the bones, and controls blood pressure. Potassium-rich foods help manage blood pressure by helping the body eliminate more sodium.

TIP: When you purchase bananas at the grocery store, look for green ones and peel them to store in your freezer. Consuming green bananas can help keep your gut bacteria healthy. It can also increase the production of short-chain fatty acids essential for digestive health.

PAPAYA

Papaya is a yellow-orange fruit with edible seeds. It contains high levels of antioxidants, vitamins A, C, and E. The high potassium content in papaya helps lower blood pressure.

TIP: Pureed papaya added to a marinade will give a tropical flavor and tenderize meat and poultry.

CANTALOUPE

The fiber, potassium, and vitamin C in cantaloupe are vital nutrients for heart health. As a good source of potassium, cantaloupe improves blood pressure and keeps the right balance between cells and body fluids.

TIP: Chopped cantaloupe is tossed with sweet cherry tomatoes, tangy red onion, and refreshing cucumber. This vibrant medley is drizzled with a zesty lime dressing to create a wonderfully delicious salad plate.

CHERRIES

Cherries are low in calories and rich in fiber, vitamins, minerals, nutrients, and other good-for-you nutrients. You'll get vitamins C, A, and K. Each long-stemmed fruit also delivers potassium, magnesium, and calcium. Cherries are also rich in antioxidants.

TIP: Cherries are delicious in salads and are nature's natural form of aspirin.

CITRUS FRUITS

Citrus fruits include lemons, limes, oranges, mandarin, and grapefruit. Citrus fruits are rich in nutrients like vitamin C, flavonoids, and fiber, offering exceptional vascular protection and reducing inflammation. Many compounds in citrus fruits can benefit heart health by improving cholesterol levels and lowering blood pressure. Citrus fruits may have powerful blood-pressure-lowering effects. They're loaded with vitamins, minerals, and plant compounds that may help keep your heart healthy by reducing heart disease risk factors like high blood pressure. A diet rich in fruits and vegetables can help you get your blood pressure under control.

TIP: Start your day by squeezing the juice of a lemon into a tall glass of water to start your day hydrated and cleanse your liver.

PEAR

Rich in fiber, natural sugar, protein, magnesium, potassium, and vitamin C, pears may lower the risk of heart disease. Their procyanidin antioxidants may decrease stiffness in heart tissue, lower LDL cholesterol, and increase HDL cholesterol. The fiber in pears may also reduce the risk of cardiovascular disease by lowering blood pressure.

TIP: Pears are an excellent fruit to keep on hand for a delicious, sweet snack.

HONEYDEW MELON

Honeydew melon is a low-sodium and potassium-rich fruit that may help maintain healthy blood pressure levels. If you want to increase your potassium intake, try adding honeydew to your diet. The potassium in honeydew counteracts the effects of sodium and relaxes blood vessel walls.

TIP: Place a peeled slice of honeydew on a plate. Pile on slices of banana and your favorite berries. Top with a scoop of fat-free frozen yogurt and a sprinkle of chopped nuts for a delicious dessert.

APPLES

Apples are high in soluble fiber, which helps lower cholesterol. The polyphenols in apples are linked to lowering blood pressure and stroke risk. Gala apples appear to prevent heart disease by reducing the main risk factors.

TIP: Enjoy an apple (preferably organic) dipped in almond butter for a delicious, energizing, satisfying snack.

GRAPES

The polyphenols in grapes, such as resveratrol, are rich in antioxidants, lipid-lowering, and anti-inflammatory actions that may help reduce the risk of cardiovascular disease. They may achieve this by preventing platelet build-up and lowering blood pressure and the risk of irregular heart rhythms.

TIP: Grapes are delicious to have on hand for a quick snack. They are also delicious in homemade chicken salad.

POMEGRANATES

Loaded with potent antioxidant and anti-inflammatory properties and other benefits, pomegranates are an effective fruit to lower blood pressure, improve HDL cholesterol, and prevent and treat plaques in the arteries that cause heart attacks and strokes.

TIP: Toss them in a green salad or sprinkle the seeds on your yogurt or oatmeal. They also add great flavor to a smoothie.

KIWI

With abundant vitamin E, C, and potassium, kiwi promotes cardiovascular health and prevents the clogging of arteries. It contains anti-inflammatory properties and fiber, which can boost heart health. Intake of two to three kiwi fruits per day can improve cardiovascular health.

TIP: Sliced kiwi is delicious in a salad or as a simple side dish for any meal.

WATERMELON

Watermelon contains three blood-pressure-supporting nutrients: L-citrulline, lycopene, and potassium. The body converts citrulline to arginine, and this helps the body produce nitric oxide. Nitric oxide relaxes blood vessels and encourages flexibility in arteries. This improves blood flow, which can lower hypertension.

TIP: Take advantage of the cut-up watermelon available in the produce section of your local grocery store, ready to eat.

CHAPTER 5

Healthy Fats

Dietary fats are essential to give your body energy and support cell function. They also help protect your organs and keep your body warm. Fats help your body absorb some nutrients and produce important hormones, too. Saturated fats raise blood cholesterol, which, like high blood pressure, can lead to heart disease and stroke. However, unsaturated fats are excellent for heart health. There are two types of unsaturated fats - polyunsaturated and mono-unsaturated fats. These are the healthiest fats for lowering blood pressure and are discussed below.

NUTS AND SEEDS

Almost all nuts (almonds, walnuts, pecans, hazelnuts, pistachios, macadamia) are packed with heart-friendly nutrients, like vitamin E, omega-3 fatty acids, fiber, and unsaturated fats. They may help fight inflammation, improve blood vessel health, and lower your risk of heart disease.

TIP: Add nuts to your favorite salad, sprinkle on your morning oatmeal or yogurt, or add to your smoothies.

AVOCADO

Avocados contain dietary fiber, unsaturated fats like monounsaturated fats, and other favorable components associated with good cardiovascular health.

TIP: Spread a small, ripe avocado on top of whole-grain toast. Season it with black pepper and sprinkle a little feta on top.

DARK CHOCOLATE

Dark chocolate contains excellent nutrients for lowering blood pressure and improving heart health. Made from the cacao tree seed, it's one of the best sources of fiber, magnesium, copper, iron, Vitamin B6, Vitamin B12, Vitamin E, Vitamin K, potassium, phosphorus, zinc, and selenium.

TIP: Stick with minimally processed dark chocolate bars that are at least 70 percent cocoa to obtain the most flavanols. Remember that the higher the percentage of cocoa, the greater the number of flavanols and the greater the bitter flavor. One ounce is all you need, about the size of your thumb.

EXTRA VIRGIN OLIVE OIL

Extra virgin olive oil is an excellent source of monounsaturated fatty acids. Research indicates that daily use of at least two tablespoons of extra virgin olive oil can lower systolic blood pressure compared to oils rich in polyunsaturated fats.

TIP: Use extra-virgin olive oil for your cooking and food preparation.

FLAXSEED

Flaxseeds are rich in Omega-3 and unsaturated fats. Flax is an excellent soluble fiber that absorbs water and slows digestion. Soluble fiber can help lower cholesterol and blood pressure.

TIP: Add ground flaxseeds to your morning smoothie or sprinkle them on salads, oatmeal, or yogurt. Ensure they are ground as the body cannot absorb their benefits in their whole state.

CHIA SEEDS

Despite their small size, chia seeds are one of the richest sources of omega-3 fatty acids, iron, calcium, and antioxidants. Chia seeds are an excellent fiber source, promoting intestinal health, improving heart health, and lowering blood pressure.

TIP: Chia seeds are versatile in recipes since they can be eaten raw, soaked in water, ground into a chia seed powder, baked into recipes, or even used as a thickening agent to replace eggs or dairy in vegan recipes.

CHAPTER 6

Proteins

Protein from various sources can help lower your risk of high blood pressure. Add seafood and legumes to your diet in addition to traditional protein sources of beef and chicken. Both plant and animal proteins are excellent at regulating blood pressure and improving heart health. Animal proteins, especially eggs, contain high arginine levels, which dilates blood vessels and lowers blood pressure. One study suggests that people with the highest protein intake—on average 102 grams daily- had a 40 percent lower risk of developing high blood pressure.

TIP: Make sure you have a protein source with every meal.

LEGUMES

Legumes are high in amino acids, fiber, and potassium. They're excellent for those with hypertension. Examples of legumes include black beans, white beans, red beans, lentils, green beans, chickpeas, and soybeans.

TIP: Make a hearty bean soup or make a bean spread. Add beans to tacos or quesadillas, or make a plant-based burger.

PASTURED EGGS

Eggs from pastured hens are reportedly more nutritious than conventional eggs. Pastured eggs are higher in vitamins A, E, and omega-3s and lower in cholesterol and saturated fat.

TIP: Always keep eggs on hand to whip up a meal anytime. A vegetable omelet is a great way to get a serving of vegetables and adds flavor.

LEAN MEAT AND STEAK

Lean grass-fed red meat is a good source of protein, omega-3 fatty acids, vitamin B12, niacin, zinc, and iron. It is trimmed of visible fat and does not increase cardiovascular risk factors.

TIP: Lean beef can be enjoyed as a protein source, along with fruits, vegetables, and low-fat dairy, to help lower blood pressure in healthy individuals.

LEAN CHICKEN

Chicken is an excellent protein source and rich in vitamins and minerals. It helps build muscles, keeps your bones strong, helps with weight loss, reduces cholesterol, and controls blood pressure.

TIP: Keep chicken breasts in hand to create a quick dinner any night of the week.

SEAFOOD

Fish and other seafood are the primary sources of healthful long-chain omega-3 fats. They also contain vitamin D, vitamin B-12, selenium, and protein. Strong evidence suggests eating fish or taking fish oil is excellent for the heart and blood vessels. Sources include shrimp, salmon, and sardines.

TIP: Incorporate seafood into your weekly menus. For example, purchase easy-peel shrimp and toss in olive oil and your favorite seafood seasoning. Grill or cook in a hot skillet for a quick meal.

PLAIN YOGURT

Plain yogurt is an excellent source of vitamin A, B12, calcium, potassium, iodine, and phosphorus. Greek yogurt's vitamins, minerals, and probiotics benefit gut and heart health. Avoid yogurt with the added fruit, as it usually contains a lot of sugar.

TIP: Create a yogurt parfait with fresh fruit, oats, and grape nuts for a delicious, filling breakfast or snack.

CHAPTER 7

Carbohydrates

Unrefined carbs and whole-grain foods are rich sources of healthy nutrients, including fiber, potassium, magnesium, folate, iron, and selenium. These nutrients are linked to lower blood pressure and reduced damage to blood vessels. The vitamins, minerals, and disease-fighting chemicals in these foods, such as phytosterols, lignans, and antioxidants, help prevent heart disease and high blood pressure.

SWEET POTATOES

Sweet potatoes are an excellent source of beta-carotene, vitamins A, C, and potassium. They are also high in fiber and antioxidants, which protect your body from free radical damage and promote a healthy gut and brain.

TIP: Substitute plain baked potato with sweet potato whenever possible. They are deliciously baked in the oven and topped with ground cinnamon, which helps stabilize blood sugar levels.

WHOLE GRAIN BREAD AND PASTA

Whole-grain bread and pasta have more fiber than regular bread and pasta. Whole grains are minimally processed, making them more nutritious than refined grains. Replacing refined grains with whole grains has been shown to lower the risk of chronic diseases like heart disease.

TIP: Look for whole-grain varieties when choosing bread or pasta at your local grocery store. You can also find pasta made from cauliflower, chickpeas, and vegetables.

BROWN RICE

Brown rice boosts heart health. It is rich in manganese, decreases cholesterol levels, and lowers diabetes risk. Brown rice provides iron to aid in oxygenating the blood and selenium, which improves blood pressure and helps to prevent heart disease.

TIP: Cook up a batch of brown rice and keep it in your refrigerator. Stir fry chicken or shrimp and vegetables, and you have a complete meal any day of the week.

QUINOA

A plant-based source of protein, quinoa is also high in antioxidants, iron, vitamin B-1, Zinc, vitamin B-6, and magnesium. Research shows that eating a diet rich in whole grains (such as quinoa and other ancient grains, oatmeal, and brown rice) helps prevent heart disease and high blood pressure.

TIP: Quinoa can be used the same way as brown rice. It has a delicious nutty flavor that enhances any dish.

WINTER SQUASH

Winter squash delivers vitamins A and C, rich in beta carotene, lutein, zeaxanthin, protein, vitamin B6, fiber, and magnesium. Butternut squash or winter squash may help prevent high blood pressure.

TIP: Some squashes—like butternut and kabocha—should be peeled before you eat them. But certain varieties, especially the smaller ones like acorn squash, have softer, more tender skins, so you don't have to bother with the peeling. Cut them in half, scoop out the seeds, and roast in the oven; cut side down in a 350-degree oven for about 40 minutes.

OATS

Oats are high in soluble fiber. The possible health benefits of oats include reducing the risk of coronary artery disease. One serving of old-fashioned oats drops blood pressure points after a few weeks.

TIP: You can make a quick snack with a container of plain yogurt, 1/3 cup of oats, cinnamon, and 2 tablespoons of raisins. Mix well and enjoy.

PLANTAINS

Plantains are a carbohydrate-rich source of fiber and essential vitamins and minerals such as folate, magnesium, vitamin C, potassium, and vitamin B6. Plantains are low in fat and sodium, and the potassium in plantains can help reduce hypertension and stroke.

TIP: Plantains are inedible raw and should be eaten only after cooking. Plantains can be prepared in numerous ways, and their flavor ranges from savory to sweet, depending on ripeness.

DATES

Dates offer significant fiber and minerals, including iron, potassium, B vitamins, copper, and magnesium. The fiber and antioxidants in dates may help protect your heart by keeping your arteries clean and reducing your risk of heart disease.

TIP: Dates are so versatile that they can be added to cakes, puddings, and biscuits or used in stews, tagines, stuffing, or salads. Or try stuffing them with ricotta or blue cheese for an elegant appetizer.

CHAPTER 8

Spices and Herbs

Herbs and spices are a fantastic addition to a healthy blood pressure diet. Some research has shown that a diet rich in herbs and spices may reduce blood pressure in people at risk of cardiovascular disease. This is excellent news! Seasoning your food with herbs and spices isn't just a way to make your meals tastier; it's also a perfect way to care for your heart health. This chapter will explore the best herbs and spices for blood pressure, specifically designed to dilate and relax the arteries.

GARLIC

Garlic is low in calories and rich in manganese. It is also rich in allicin and alliinase, which help boost the immune system and lower high blood pressure and LDL cholesterol levels.

TIP: When you smash and chop fresh garlic for recipes, get the most goodness out of your allicin by leaving the prepared garlic for ten minutes – so just as you would let a good wine breathe, leave your garlic to rest before adding it to the pan or recipe.

TURMERIC

Curcumin is turmeric's main ingredient, with powerful antioxidant and anti-inflammatory properties. Studies suggest that turmeric contains bioactive compounds that activate the body's antibody responses and combat chronic diseases like heart disease.

TIP: When adding fresh turmeric to a recipe, you'll probably want to cook it rather than serve it raw. Raw turmeric can have a strong, pungent flavor but mellows as it cooks.

GINGER

Gingerol, a bioactive compound found in ginger, is antimicrobial and anti-fungal. Ginger contains antioxidants and is anti-inflammatory; ginger helps with digestion and gut health, which impact heart health. It is also a good source of vitamin C, magnesium, potassium, copper, and manganese. Ginger helps lower and keep your blood vessels supple and dilated.

TIP: Once peeled and grated, ginger can easily be thrown into various sauces, glazes, and marinades to brighten the dish.

CEYLON CINNAMON

Cinnamon is an excellent source of antioxidants, and as is true for many spices, cinnamon provides delicious nutrition without calories. It improves blood flow, stimulates circulation, lowers blood sugar, and protects against diabetes, decreasing the risk of heart attacks and strokes.

TIP: Start your day with half a teaspoon of ground cinnamon in your morning coffee. It adds great flavor and helps stabilize blood sugar levels for the day.

CAYENNE PEPPER

Cayenne pepper is a good source of antioxidants, vitamin C, vitamin A, vitamin B6, vitamin K, and a special plant compound called capsaicin. Capsaicin protects cells, improves digestion, and maintains a healthy weight. Based on studies, capsaicin may help to reduce high blood pressure.

TIP: Keep cayenne pepper spice on hand to add to your favorite recipes. Given its high heat levels, cayenne is best used in small amounts while cooking to guarantee that this concentrated spice doesn't overtake a dish.

FRESH HERBS

Fresh herbs include basil, cilantro, dill, mint, oregano, parsley, rosemary, thyme, and sage. These herbs contain vitamins C, A, and B, iron, magnesium, and manganese. Various herbs have been shown to give your heart an additional health boost.

TIP: Add some loose leaves to boiling water and sip as tea, or add to stews, soups, and salads. Start an herb garden to enjoy your favorite freshest of herbs.

Herbs and spices make food tastier while boosting your health. Cook with herbs and spices regularly. Use several at a time for maximum health benefits.

CHAPTER 9
BEVERAGES

The right beverage can work wonders to improve blood pressure. When a person has high blood pressure, every beverage you drink should dilate, relax, and nourish your arteries. Below are a few of the best liquids that hydrate for proper heart functioning and improve arterial blood flow.

WATER

Chronic dehydration raises blood pressure levels by making the body hold on to sodium. Keeping the body hydrated helps the heart pump blood to the muscles and other organs. 2-3 liters of water daily is ideal.

TIP: Invest in a water bottle you can keep throughout your day. Jazz it up with some fresh lemon slices for added flavor.

TEA

Tea is full of heart-healthy compounds that help fight inflammation and cell damage. Black and green tea, dandelion, and hibiscus tea are associated with a lower risk of heart attack and stroke; short-term studies suggest they're good for your blood vessel health.

TIP: Explore the tea section at your local health food or grocery store and enjoy a cup of tea in the afternoon.

RED WINE

In moderation, red wine has long been considered healthy for the heart. Polyphenols and antioxidants in red wine may help prevent coronary artery disease. You can avoid wine if you don't drink alcohol. There are plenty of other food options in this book.

TIP: If you are not a wine drinker, consider taking resveratrol as a supplement or eat red grapes to reap the many health benefits.

JUICING

Juicing prevents hardening of the arteries, lowers cholesterol, and decreases blood pressure. For maximum nutrients, juice a variety of vegetables and fruits. Specifically, beetroot juice is popular due to its high nitrate content, which widens blood vessels.

TIP: Invest in a juicer that will allow you to get in the habit of juicing regularly. Find one that is easy to use and clean. Good choices of food to juice include beets, carrots, celery, and apples.

HERB-INFUSED WATER

Herb-infused water is rich in vitamins and minerals. Its benefits include appetite control, hydration, heartburn prevention, blood sugar regulation, and weight management. Infuse your water with herbs like sage, thyme, and rosemary. Enjoy!

TIP: Infuse a pitcher of ice-cold water with herbs and store it in your refrigerator for a hydration treat.

Beverages to Avoid

Just as some drinks can help lower blood pressure, others may increase blood pressure levels. Here are some drinks that you may need to limit or avoid if you have high blood pressure:

Soft Drinks

Most soft drinks with added sugar can significantly increase your risk for heart disease and high blood pressure. Did you know your body does not like soft drinks? Drinking soda is bad for your health in so many ways that science cannot even begin to state ALL the consequences to your health. Here is what happens in your body when you assault it with a Coke:

Within the first 10 minutes – 10 teaspoons of sugar hit your system – this is 100% of your recommended daily intake. The ONLY reason you do not vomit due to the overwhelming sweetness is that phosphoric acid cuts the sweetness. Unfortunately, phosphoric acid BLOCKS the absorption of calcium in your bones.

Within 20 minutes – your blood sugar spikes, and your liver responds to the insulin burst by turning massive amounts of sugar into fat.

Within 40 minutes – caffeine absorption is complete – your pupils dilate, blood pressure rises, and your liver dumps more sugar into your bloodstream.

About 45 minutes later – your body increases dopamine production, which stimulates the pleasure centers of the brain – which is the physically identical response to heroin.

After One Hour – you will start to have a blood sugar crash and likely reach for another Coke or another source of sugar or caffeine. If you do, the vicious cycle continues.

DIET SOFT DRINKS have many other problems related to artificial sweeteners because they promote hunger. Why? The brain registers that you received something sweet – however, your stomach says, "where is it?" This is why many people report feeling hungry within an hour of consuming a diet soft drink.

Getting off soft drinks can be challenging, so try this tactic – get your soft drink and get a nice tall glass of ice water. Jazz it up with some lemon. Drink a few sips of soft drink and a few sips of water – do it again! Eventually, your body will tell you that water feels better, allowing you to wean yourself off soft drinks. Invest in a water bottle so it is easy to keep water with you at all times, whether at home or work.

Sweetened Beverages

Like soda, other sweetened drinks, such as iced tea, are packed with sugar. Iced tea is one of the most commonly consumed sugar-sweetened beverages in the United States. Choose unsweetened tea whenever possible to limit your sugar intake and avoid a negative effect on your blood pressure.

Energy drinks

In addition to providing a concentrated amount of caffeine and added sugar in each serving, research shows that certain energy drinks can significantly increase your systolic and diastolic blood pressure levels.

Alcohol

Some research suggests that even moderate amounts of alcohol may be linked to high blood pressure. If you drink alcohol, talk to your doctor to determine whether lowering your intake is necessary.

CHAPTER 10

Supplement Your Diet

Supplements are exactly that – they supplement a healthy diet. There is a prevalent misconception that supplements (or a specific supplement) can lower blood pressure. This belief has led many people to frustrating outcomes because this isn't true. Supplements should be taken as part of a healthy lifestyle.

A supplement contains one or more dietary ingredients, including vitamins, minerals, herbs, and amino acids. It is intended to be taken by mouth and is labeled on the front panel as a dietary supplement. Dietary supplements can also be extracts or concentrates and may be found in various forms, such as pills, capsules, soft gels, gel caps, liquids, or powders.

Dietary supplements are very popular. During 2017–2018, 57.6% of American adults took one form of dietary supplement or the other, and the percentage of adults using dietary supplements increased with age. Multivitamin-mineral supplements are the most commonly taken dietary supplements, followed by vitamin D, magnesium, and omega-3 fatty acid products.

Vitamin D3 + K2

While vitamin D3 increases calcium levels, vitamin K2 helps the body use it by moving it into your bones. Increasing your intake of vitamin D3 without enough vitamin K2 can cause an increase in calcium levels in the blood without the ability to use it effectively, which raises the risk of depositing calcium in arteries and soft tissue.

Therefore, vitamin D3 and vitamin K2 must be taken together. Supplementing these vitamins helps the body use calcium properly to build bone instead of depositing it dangerously in arteries and soft tissue. Vitamin K has a protective effect on arteries, preventing buildup and therefore protecting against cardiovascular disease.

Omega-3

An important supplement for everyone is fish oil, which contains an omega-3 fatty acid that can help with everything from cardiovascular health and brain functioning to arthritis and inflammation. People are encouraged to eat cold-water fatty fish, like salmon, sardines, herring, anchovies, trout, and mackerel, twice a week. The reality, however, is that people are not eating enough fish, so fish oil supplements are necessary.

Multivitamin

Multivitamins contain a combination of vitamins and minerals, and they are generally considered safe for most people when taken at recommended doses. For individuals with hypertension or at risk of developing high blood pressure, be cautious about the sodium and potassium content in multivitamins, as some multivitamin supplements may contain sodium, which can contribute to high blood pressure in sensitive individuals.

Magnesium

You need magnesium for many bodily tasks. It is involved in more than 300 chemical reactions in the body. Muscles require magnesium to contract; nerves need it to send and receive messages. It keeps your heart beating steadily and your immune system robust. Most people can get enough magnesium by eating green leafy vegetables, whole grains, beans, nuts, and fish.

Even with an adequate diet, some people are at increased risk of magnesium deficiency, and in these situations, magnesium supplements may be necessary. Magnesium isn't just good for your physical health. It is also essential for your mental well-being. Your stress levels, mood, and sleep quality are deeply linked to magnesium. For example, magnesium helps regulate our stress-response systems. It also increases levels of GABA, a neurochemical that encourages deep sleep and relaxation. Supplemental magnesium can improve sleep, reduce stress, and bring greater calm.

A Final Word on Supplements

Maintaining good heart health, especially regarding eating habits, can sometimes be challenging. Many of us struggle to eat our recommended daily portions of fruits and vegetables, whole grains, and lean proteins, all of which comprise a healthy and health-preserving diet. Whether it's because we feel we're too busy to eat a well-rounded meal before starting our day, or simply because we've never really developed the urge for smoothies, or the discipline to stick to an optimal diet plan, a safe way out is to fill any nutritional gaps with vitamins and supplements. Yet, we must ensure we take these supplements as safely as possible.

Shop my favorite brand of supplements at:

www.nicolineambe.com/shop

EAT TO LOWER BLOOD PRESSURE

GROCERY SHOPPING LIST FOR HIGH BP

Vegetables	Fruits	Healthy Fats
· Cabbage	· Berries	· Avocado
· Broccoli	· Banana	· Dark chocolate
· Cauliflower	· Papaya	· Olive oil
· Kale	· Cantaloupe	. Nuts and seeds
· Beetroot	· Cherries	. Fatty fish
· Celery	· Citrus fruits	
· Carrots	· Pears	**Nuts and Seeds**
· Chard	· Honeydew melon	· Walnuts
· Tomatoes	· Watermelon	· Almonds
· Brussel sprouts	· Apples	· Pistachios
· Onions	· Grapes	· Flaxseed
· Leeks	· Pomegranates	· Chia seeds
· Arugula	· Kiwi	. Hempseed
· Dandelion greens	. Peaches	. Pumpkin Seeds
· Artichokes	. Mangos	. Cashews
· Collard greens	. Oranges	. Sunflower seeds
· Beet greens	. Pineapple	. Brazil nuts
· Spinach	. Plum	. Peanuts
. Green beans	. Apricots	. Pecans
. Lettuce		. Macadamia
. Asparagus		
Proteins	**Beverages**	**Carbohydrates**
· Legumes	· Water	· Sweet potatoes
· Pastured eggs	· Tea	· Potatoes
· Lean meats and steak	· Red wine	· Brown rice
· Lean chicken	· Fruits for juicing	· Quinoa
· Seafood	· Herb-infused water	· Winter squash
· Plain, non-fat yogurt	· Beet juice	· Oats
. Beans	. Lemon Water	· Plantain
. Lentils	· Hot Cocoa	· Dates
. Peanut butter	. Apple cider water	. Whole Wheat Pasta
. Tempeh	· Pomegranate Juice	. Starchy vegetables
. Edamame		. Whole wheat bread

63

SUPPLEMENT YOUR DIET

Spices	**Fresh Herbs**	**Supplements**
· Garlic	· Rosemary	· Vitamin D3+K2
· Turmeric	· Parsley	· Omega-3
· Ginger	· Dill	· Magnesium
· **Ceylon** Cinnamon	· Cilantro	· Multivitamin
· Cayenne pepper	· Oregano	
	· Mint	Shop supplements at:
	· Thyme	nicolineambe.com/shop
	· Sage	
	· Basil	

CONCLUSION
Toxin-free food

Here is a quick summary of the basics of eating to lower blood pressure:

- Eat more fish, nuts, and legumes.
- Turn to vegetables and fruits instead of sugary or salty snacks and desserts.
- Select bread, pasta, and other carbohydrate-rich foods made from whole grains instead of highly refined white flour.
- Eat fruit instead of drinking fruit juice.
- Use unsaturated fats like olive oil instead of butter.
- Rely on fresh foods instead of canned and processed foods.
- Use herbs, spices, and other low-sodium flavorings instead of salt.
- Try to burn at least as many calories each day as you take in.

Proper diet and exercise can control the condition and limit symptoms for many people with hypertension or high blood pressure. A healthy eating plan including nutrients that improve heart health and blood flow can reduce the need for medication and lower the risk of heart disease or stroke.

There isn't one single "magic" food that lowers blood pressure. Instead, it is all about finding an all-around healthy eating strategy that works for you, is good for blood pressure, and offers good health.

We often overcomplicate diet by subscribing to miracle food and fad diet plans. Yet, eating healthily is fundamentally very simple. I would summarize the entire concept in three short sentences:

Eat food. Eat a reasonable amount. Eat organically.

As far as supplements are concerned, they're not food either. The average American spends $56 on nutritional supplements every month. If you eat the right food, that may be $56 too much. Many supplements can be ineffective at best and, at worst, may even be ultimately detrimental to overall well-being. The constituents of these supplements are not always controlled. They are not drugs that are subjected to intensive clinical trials, meaning they don't come under serious control by health agencies.

Medical science accepts that multivitamin pills don't act in your body like when you ingest them directly from plants. This is because utterly different chemical processes are taking place in both situations. We love the idea of a simple pill to solve all our health problems. Unfortunately, life is not that simple. Nothing worthwhile comes without the investment of time and effort.

It would be best if you approached healthy eating from an organic perspective. That said, some excellent supplements have been shown to deliver optimum benefits. As you get older, your health should be a priority. You cannot do the same things you did as a younger man or woman. Your body is changing, losing valuable minerals needed for optimum health. I wasn't aware of this until I became very ill. I struggled with many debilitating health issues for several years, including high blood pressure, heart disease, tinnitus, leg and back pain, digestive problems, hormonal imbalance, and sleep disorder.

It wasn't until I drastically changed my diet and added more plants and nutrients to my regimen that I started on the path to complete healing. I do not wish to see any man or woman endure a life of sluggishness, sickness, or even confusion about available wellness options. Be empowered to improve the quality of your life through education on nutrient-dense foods and supplements packed with powerful vitamins and minerals. Changing what you put in your mouth will improve your health. It will also prevent disease. You will enjoy increased endurance, immune support, improved sexual health, and better weight management.

Live Toxin-Free

An important aspect of being healthier is removing toxins from your diet. You are not alone in the battle against toxins. I've had my fair share of toxins in my body, and that personal experience has revealed that toxins harm our bodies in more ways than we can see. The result of long-standing exposure to toxins is chronic diseases, mild to severe health issues, and general malaise like fatigue. Removing toxins from your body gives your cells, DNA, and hormones room to breathe.

However, when you first start, toxin-free living can be overwhelming. It would seem as though everything you know and love is wrong for your health. In this simple guide, I will ease you gently into a toxin-free existence and help provide a realistic balance, but first, here are some ways toxins are harmful:

- Toxins damage your DNA, which increases your rate of aging and degeneration.
- Toxins interfere with your hormones and cause hormonal imbalance.
- Toxins displace your structural minerals.

These are some of the toxins to watch out for:

- White Table Salt
- Excessive Alcohol
- Cigarette Smoke
- Narcotics

- Refined sugar
- Soda and sports drinks
- Greasy, fatty, or processed foods
- Environmental toxins

Non-Toxic Living Starts with A Mindset

When it comes to non-toxic living, start small and work your way to completely understand how harmful food and toxic environmental chemicals have crept into your life. If you try to take everything at once, you will almost certainly feel so exasperated that you may want to give up. Yet, the non-toxic lifestyle is worth the effort. It is an investment in your future. Therefore, eliminating toxins from your food and environment is a journey, not a destination.

Most unlikely, you will wake up tomorrow and find that you have successfully replaced your entire space with organic food and chemical-free products. To transition to clean living, start with the right mindset and become a researcher in your daily life, seeking the truth about what is toxic and not toxic to you. Every new thing you bring into your home and your body should be evaluated for safety. Each time you replace something harmful with something safe, you move your toxic meter's needle in the right direction. Your body is resilient. It is designed to heal.

Your goal should be to eliminate as many toxins as you can. One of the biggest repositories of toxins is our food. In conventional farming, the food we eat is sprayed with pesticides and other chemicals that are harmful to human health. The animals that provide our meat also feed on food sprayed with chemicals. Furthermore, genetically modified plants have entered our food system. Be a vigilant and discerning consumer.

Eat Organic Food

Although organic food is more expensive, it is better for your health. Buy local produce whenever possible or grow your food. Buying locally doesn't guarantee that toxic chemicals aren't being sprayed on your food, but it is easier to find out when you can talk to the farmer.

Organically grown food has 60% more nutrients than conventionally grown food. There are also significantly lower levels of heavy metals in organic crops. The most common way we get exposed to pesticides is through food. Chronic exposure to pesticides is associated with respiratory problems, memory disorders, skin conditions, depression, miscarriage, congenital disabilities, cancer, and neurological conditions such as Parkinson's disease. Most processed foods are made with wheat, so avoiding processed foods can reduce exposure.

Add More Plants to Your Diet

The best source of vitamins and minerals is real food. Plants contain many of the nutrients we need in a form that our bodies can digest and absorb. Adding more fruits and vegetables to your diet is a way to get vitamins and minerals.

Consider Fresh Herbs

Often, our bodies need extra help and support. Herbs can be an excellent, all-natural way to improve your health. Herbs also add great flavor to meals without having to add much salt. It is highly beneficial to use fresh herbs daily in moderate quantities, as they are packed with many health-boosting compounds. This is the foundation of the Mediterranean diet. Pesto, for example, uses basil as its base with plenty of garlic, both of which offer significant nutritional benefits for heart health and blood pressure.

Pay Attention to Your Supplements

Pay attention to what ingredients are in your supplements. It is important to know the composition of a supplement and where it comes from. Is the supplement from a whole food source or an inorganic source? Does it come from the United States or another country? What kinds of fillers or preservatives does it have? What conditions do you intend the supplement to resolve?

TWO MONTHS BLOOD PRESSURE ROUTINE

This is the exact 2-month routine I used (and still use) to lower my blood pressure with whole foods, lifestyle medication, and effective supplementation. It requires discipline and consistency.

WEEK ONE

Every morning this week, upon rising, sip one liter of warm lemon water with 1/2 or 1 whole squeezed lemon. This helps detoxify your body and prepare your gut to absorb nutrients.

Eat your first regular healthy meal at 12 noon. If applicable, take any medications at that time as well. Intermittent fasting helps to lower blood pressure, reduce inflammation, improve insulin sensitivity, and lower cholesterol.

Take your blood pressure reading daily when you wake up, then retake it later.

Taking your blood pressure readings daily helps you understand your blood pressure patterns – what makes it rise and what lowers it. You also monitor your progress so that you can adjust your routines and lifestyle to achieve your desired blood pressure goals.

This week, find 10 minutes every day to take deep breaths, reduce anxiety, eliminate stress, and calm your heart. Did you know 30% of people have high blood pressure due to anxiety? Let's breathe!

WEEK TWO

Maintain your routine from week 1.

You will be challenged a little this week. Be inspired and excited, not anxious, or fearful :)

This week, add a finger-pinch of organic cayenne pepper to your lemon water. Add just enough cayenne to color your water. It should NOT be spicy to the taste.

Also, this week, chew one small clove of raw garlic first thing in the morning BEFORE your lemon/cayenne water. This detoxifies your intestines, improves circulation, lowers inflammation, stabilizes your blood pressure, and feeds your good gut bacteria for improved nutrient absorption. (Chewing is better)

This week, order your supplements and other products needed in the program. Order them from my website at **www.nicolineambe.com/shop** or your local Whole Foods store. You will need them in week four. ***See the shopping list below.***

When you order from my website, your products will ship from Amazon. (I earn a small commission)

EAT TO LOWER BLOOD PRESSURE

Product list to order

- Omega 3 fish oil or Plant-based omega-3
- Magnesium Glycinate
- Vitamin D3+K2
- Multivitamin
- Hawthorn Berry
- Extra Virgin Olive Oil
- Plant-based Protein (for more protein - Optional)
- Organic Cayenne Pepper
- Organic Chia Seed
- Organic Flaxseed
- Nutribullet for smoothie
- Green Tea
- Apple Cider Vinegar
- Non-stick air fryer

Every day this week, do a 30-minute workout on YouTube or go for a brisk walk.

Order your products from **www.nicolineambe.com/shop**.

WEEK THREE

Maintain your routine from weeks 1 and 2

Here are your options for 12 noon after your fast.

OPTION 1 - Make a small fruit bowl. Wash your fruits clean. Add 5 of the fruits below to your fruit bowl.

- Papaya
- Blueberries
- Raspberries
- Strawberries
- Cantaloupe
- Kiwi
- Apple
- Peach
- Grapes
- Pear
- Dragon fruit

Add any of the following healthy fats to your fruit bowl.

1. Avocado
2. Nuts and seeds.
3. OR eat one tablespoon of organic extra virgin olive oil before you eat your fruit.

(The fruit option is my preferred option)

EAT TO LOWER BLOOD PRESSURE

OPTION 2 - Make a small bowl of whole-grain Quaker oats. Add the following:

- Quaker Oats - 100% whole grain old fashioned oats
- Top it with blueberries, raspberries, strawberries, and a pinch of Ceylon cinnamon.
- Use one cup of non-fat, sugar-free whole milk OR one cup of almond milk OR plain water (preferably) to prepare your oats.
- Side of 1 cup of non-fat, sugar-free Greek yogurt
- Side of 1 hard-boiled egg or 2 egg whites
- Serve with green tea or black tea. Use monk fruit or raw honey to sweeten your oat or tea (optional).
- Eat one tablespoon of organic extra virgin olive oil before eating oatmeal.
- Exercise EVERY DAY this week. Find 30 minutes in your day to exercise. Use any YouTube video OR go for a 30-minute brisk walk.

WEEK FOUR

Week 4: Make a Nutrient-Dense Smoothie

Maintain your routines from weeks 1, 2, and 3.

NOTE--> THIS IS THE MOST CHALLENGING WEEK IN THE PROGRAM BUT ALSO THE MOST IMPORTANT!

2 MONTHS BLOOD PRESSURE ROUTINE

One of the things that will separate you from people who continue to struggle with high blood pressure and other health issues is how much nutrients you eat. The leading cause of disease is nutrient deficiency. People are not eating enough nutrients.

NUTRITION IS KEY!

This week, you will add a nutrient-dense veggie smoothie to your routine. A smoothie is the best way to pack many healthy veggies for more nutrients. Wash your veggies with salt, vinegar, OR baking soda. Make a deluxe combo smoothie with ALL the ingredients listed below...

Add small amounts of ALL these veggies.

ADD a handful of leafy greens - kale, spinach, chard, arugula, collards, Bok choy, and dandelion. (Choose 3 from this list every week.)

ADD cruciferous vegetables (Red cabbage, green cabbage, broccoli, asparagus, Brussels sprouts, zucchini, carrots. (Choose 3 from this list every week)

<u>Also, add the following to your veggie smoothie.</u>

- Beetroot
- Raw turmeric root
- Raw ginger root
- Raw garlic clove
- Avocado

- 1tbs flaxseed
- 1tbs chia seed
- 5 raw walnuts
- 5 raw almonds
- 5 raw pistachios
- 10 pumpkin seeds
- One scoop of whey protein powder (Optional)

How to sweeten your veggie smoothie

- One whole banana
- Organic dried raisins to taste (optional)
- Organic dried cranberries to taste (optional)
- 1 pitted Medjool date (Optional)
- Raw organic honey

Fill your blender with the desired amount of filtered water and/or 1/4 cup of coconut water for more potassium (Optional) - Use natural coconuts (if possible)

DO NOT add fruit to your smoothie except bananas.

REMEMBER... Only add small amounts of each veggie to make one serving. Make it palatable to your taste buds and how you like it. DO NOT SAVE SMOOTHIE FOR FUTURE USE.

Blend everything with water and/or organic coconut water until creamy. Enjoy! :)

Take these supplements with your smoothie.

- 1 Omega-3 fish oil
- 1 Vitamin D3+K2
- 1 multivitamin.
- 1 Hawthorn berry (optional)

NOTE: *Veggie smoothie is high in fiber. Fiber takes a long time to digest. So, you will feel full. Sip green tea to move fiber quicker along your digestive tract or stay physically active.*

Exercise every day this week. Find 30 minutes in your day to exercise. Use any YouTube video OR go for a brisk 30-minute walk.

Take 1 magnesium glycinate and 1 hawthorn berry with your last meal in the evening. Follow with plain water.

WEEK FIVE

Week 5: Eat a Healthy Meal OR a Rainbow Salad

Maintain your routines from weeks 1, 2, 3, 4.

This week, after your smoothie, you get to enjoy a healthy cooked meal. After your smoothie, eat a warm meal OR make a protein-rich rainbow salad. Prepare your meals with ANY of the food options listed below. Use your favorite recipes. The key is to ensure that you are eating meals that are healthy for you.

Eat your last meal before 7 pm or at least 2 HOURS BEFORE bed.

EAT TO LOWER BLOOD PRESSURE

OPTION 1: HEALTHY MEAL

Protein

- Beans
- Green beans
- Lean pastured chicken
- Lean meat/steak
- Freshwater fish
- Eggs

Carbohydrate

- Brown rice
- Sweet potatoes
- Winter squash
- Quinoa
- Whole grain pasta

Vegetable

Cruciferous vegetables (Broccoli, cauliflower, asparagus, cabbage, Arugula, and Brussels sprout)

Leafy green vegetables (Kale, chard, spinach, collards, turnips, Bok choy)

Seasoning

- Fresh herbs (basil, cilantro, rosemary, thyme)
- Cayenne pepper (if you like spicy food)
- Leeks and green onions

- Garlic, onion, tomatoes
- Sodium-free dried seasoning
- Yellow, red, orange, and green bell peppers
- Cooking oil will be a choice of olive, avocado, or coconut oil. Olive oil is preferred.

Dessert

- Enjoy your favorite low-sugar dessert or dark chocolate with 90-100% cocoa.
- If you drink alcohol, enjoy a 5 oz glass of red wine with your meal or enjoy some green tea

OPTION 2: RAINBOW SALAD

Use the following in your rainbow salad.

- Leafy greens
- Romaine or butter lettuce
- Beans
- Onions
- Berries
- Mushrooms
- Raw nuts and seeds (walnuts, pumpkin, almonds, pistachios)
- Your favorite homemade salad dressing

Exercise every day this week. Use a YouTube video with 3-10-pound weights for toning, or go for a brisk walk.

EAT TO LOWER BLOOD PRESSURE

WEEK SIX

Drink a Blood Pressure-lowering beverage.

Maintain your routines from weeks 1, 2, 3, 4 and 5.

This week, after your lemon/cayenne water and smoothie, you will add another healthy beverage to your routine. What you drink is just as important as what you eat. Here are your options for beverages that lower blood pressure.

OPTION 1: Herb-infused Water

- Fresh Mint
- Fresh Rosemary
- Fresh Thyme

Pour water into a one-liter insulated bottle. Add cinnamon stick (optional). Wash your preferred herb combo and add to your water. Let it sit in the refrigerator for at least 20 minutes. Sip throughout the day. You may also add other veggies like cucumber.

OPTION 2: FRESH Juice (Juicing)

- Beetroot
- Ginger
- Celery OR carrot OR both
- Apples (Green or red)

Wash the veggies above and juice them. Pour the juice into a glass. Sip and enjoy!

2 MONTHS BLOOD PRESSURE ROUTINE

OPTION 3: Apple Cider Vinegar Water

Pour water into your liter bottle. Add 1-2 capfuls of Apple Cider Vinegar (The Mother) into your bottle. Add half a lemon (optional). Sip after your smoothie.

OPTION 4: Drink Tea (best before 4 pm)

Sip a liter of green tea, dandelion tea, or hibiscus tea.

Add your preferred tea to a liter of hot, warm, cool, or cold water. Sip and enjoy! Drink your tea before 4 pm as tea may contain a certain amount of caffeine. Make sure you purchase quality teas.

OPTION 5: Add Saffron to water.

Add 5-7 threads of saffron to one liter of water. Add cinnamon (optional). Let it sit for 30 minutes. Then add green tea (optional). Sip and enjoy!

OPTION 6: Ginger/Turmeric Tea

In the evening, make ginger/turmeric tea. Blend raw ginger and raw turmeric in your nutribullet. Pour it into a pot. Add water and boil for one minute. Turn off the stove and strain it into a teacup. Add 1 tablespoon of raw honey. Relax. Sip. Enjoy!

OPTION 7: Ceylon Cinnamon and Lemon

Add Ceylon Cinnamon Stick and half a lemon to a liter of cold/cool/warm water. Sip and enjoy through the afternoon.

WEEK SEVEN

Breathe, Meditate, and Sleep

Maintain your routines from Weeks 1, 2, 3, 4, 5, and 6.

Staying very relaxed is a crucial part of maintaining normal blood pressure. Stress, nervousness, anxiety, or unease are enemies of your blood pressure. You must LEARN TO BREATHE, RELAX, AND REMAIN CALM AT ALL TIMES. There are three important ways to stay calm. These are by practicing breathwork, meditation, and quality sleep. Here's how to practice them this week.

Breathe

EVERY DAY this week, take 5 minutes to practice deep breathing. If you have ever felt like your breathing is shallow and you can't breathe in enough air, here is a simple technique to help you breathe deeply, relax your body, and lower your blood pressure. Breathing deeply can also positively affect your mental and physical health. It can boost your energy levels, reduce stress and anxiety, and help you sleep better.

Start by sitting in a comfortable position with your back straight. Close your eyes and take a few deep breaths through your nose and out through your nose or mouth.

Focus your attention on the way the air moves in and out of your body. Feel your chest and belly gently expanding and contracting. Stay completely relaxed.

As you continue to breathe, take deeper breaths. Inhale slowly through your nose and count to four. Exhale through your mouth and count to five.

To deepen your breath even more, place one hand on your stomach and the other on your chest. As you breathe in, imagine your stomach expanding like a balloon. As you exhale, feel it gently deflate.

Continue to breathe this way for a few minutes until you feel like you're in deep ease and relaxation.

Taking the time to breathe deeply can help ease tension and relax your body. Try it out a few times daily and see how much better you feel.

Meditate

Find 10 minutes every day this week to meditate. Set an intention for what you want to draw into your life. Find a gentle meditation video on YouTube or in your App Store that is soothing and helps you reconcile any parts of you that are anxious, concerned, or tense. Use it to acknowledge those emotions and let them go.

Just for this moment, let go of all worries, concerns, and issues that rob you of your well-being and normal blood pressure.

Clear your mind, quiet your heart, and find balance.

Sleep

Get 7-9 hours of quality sleep every night. Here are a few sleep tips.

- Wear socks on your feet (if you're cold)

- Remove noise and internet/social media browsing from your bedroom.

- Mindfully release all worries while you sleep. Let them go so you can heal. Unclench your jaws and take relaxing breaths while you sleep.

- To further relax, do light stretches and breathing exercises before bed. This will relax you and improve your breathing to lower blood pressure.

WEEK EIGHT

Week 8: Tips to lower your BP throughout the day.

Maintain your routines from weeks 1, 2, 3, 4, 5, 6, 7

Every 2 hours, you should eat, drink, do breathwork, or exercise to keep your blood pressure normal. Here are some ways to implement the 2-hour rule.

- Eat one raw garlic clove first thing in the morning.
- Sip lemon/cayenne water in the morning until 12 noon
- Eat your heart-healing fruit or oatmeal bowl with any healthy fat – avocado, olive oil, or nuts.

2 MONTHS BLOOD PRESSURE ROUTINE

- Eat your nutrient-dense smoothie. Take your one-a-day multivitamin, Vitamin D3+K2, and Omega-3
- Sip your second liter of blood-pressure-lowering beverage.
- Exercise for at least 30 minutes daily. Stay in motion and physically active throughout the day.
- Stay relaxed and practice deep, relaxing breathing for 5-10 minutes daily.
- Eat a heart-healthy, cooked meal, OR enjoy a rainbow salad after your smoothie.
- Take your magnesium glycinate and hawthorn berry supplements with your last meal in the evening.
- No food after 7 pm. The fasting window opens.
- Enjoy good quality sleep for 7-8 hours. Breathe and stay relaxed as you sleep.
- Check your blood pressure daily and consult with your doctor.

TRACK YOUR FOOD INTAKE

Now that you have a general idea of what to eat and how to combine foods to improve heart health and lower blood pressure, I invite you to track your weekly food intake. During the next seven weeks, write down everything you eat during the day. Be mindful of controlling your portions to avoid extra calories that can cause weight gain. Also, keep track of your progress with a blood pressure log, weigh yourself often, and take before/after pictures. This will help you adjust as you go so you can achieve your desired goal. If you don't already have a blood pressure logbook, you can order one from **www.nicolineambe.com/books**

FOOD DIARY – WEEK ONE

Week of _____

MORNING

BREAKFAST

LUNCH

SNACKS

DINNER

DRINKS

PROGRESS

FOOD DIARY – WEEK TWO

Week of: _____

MORNING

BREAKFAST

LUNCH

SNACKS

DINNER

DRINKS

PROGRESS

FOOD DIARY – WEEK THREE

Week of:_____

MORNING

BREAKFAST

LUNCH

SNACKS

DINNER

DRINKS

PROGRESS

FOOD DIARY – WEEK FOUR

Week of: _____

MORNING

BREAKFAST

LUNCH

SNACKS

DINNER

DRINKS

PROGRESS

FOOD DIARY – WEEK FIVE

Week of:_____

MORNING

BREAKFAST

LUNCH

SNACKS

DINNER

DRINKS

PROGRESS

FOOD DIARY – WEEK SIX

Week of:_____

MORNING

BREAKFAST

LUNCH

SNACKS

DINNER

DRINKS

PROGRESS

FOOD DIARY – WEEK SEVEN

Week of:_____

MORNING

BREAKFAST

LUNCH

SNACKS

DINNER

DRINKS

PROGRESS

PRAISE FOR EAT TO LOWER BLOOD PRESSURE

My name is Mirabelle Beck. I am a Family Nurse Practitioner and mother. Being pregnant with my daughter left me with hypertension. Even as a practitioner, I tried all I knew but continued to struggle with the numbers. Family genetics made this challenge harder. In my practice, hypertension and its complications remain a daily educational topic for my patients in the office. Every time I educate my patients on the complications of hypertension, such as aneurysms, heart failure, kidney disease, eye problems, dementia, etc., it resonates within me because I was psychologically and physiologically paralyzed by the same. With so much information out there and many food items loaded with artificial substances and chemicals, knowing precisely what was good and not was challenging even for a practitioner. I tried to stick with the fifth-grader approach of "if I cannot read it, I will not eat it."

After over a year of struggling with the condition, I joined Dr. Nicoline Ambe Franklin's five-day eating challenge! It not only challenged me, but it also changed my life! The plan was straightforward, integrative, and simple to follow. All the food items were available; the best part was that there were no unidentifiable words. She put the plan together, and I had to follow and use the substitution she made available. Not only did I lose weight, but my blood pressure is now controlled, I am off medications, and my body glows. I integrated this into my practice and part of the management plan for hypertension, and my patients are beside themselves and grateful for their new, improved numbers and health.

See more client testimonials at:

www.nicolineambe.com/clients

LAST WORDS

I hope you have found this book helpful. The ideas contained in this book are the exact strategies I used to overcome high blood pressure and all my health issues. This is the same information I use to coach my clients who desire to lower their blood pressure. The routines are probably not how you are accustomed to living daily. However, to change something, you must do things differently than you've always done. Managing high blood pressure requires skill, consistency, precision, and commitment. It takes hard work. High blood pressure is not an easy condition to beat. If your health is important to you and if you desire to blossom as you age, then do what it takes - *read the information with careful eyes and stick to the routines.*

I am always available to support you. If you desire one-on-one coaching, reach out to me at **www.nicolincambc.com/coaching.**

STAY IN TOUCH

If you own a copy of this book, I invite you to subscribe to my newsletter at **www.nicolineambe.com**. Scroll to the bottom of the page and enter your name and email. I also invite you to join my Blood Pressure Coaching Program, which will help you apply the ideas in this book more practically and effectively. You will also have access to me for questions, check-ins, and follow-ups to ensure your blood pressure readings meet your desired goal. While your personal information will be kept private, the coaching group will allow you to interact with others who have similar struggles and are winning the battle against high blood pressure. The link to join the coaching program is **www.nicolineambe.com/coaching**

ABOUT THE AUTHOR

Nicoline Ambe is a Holistic Wellness Educator, Health Coach, entrepreneur, and Inspirational Speaker. Nicoline is passionate about helping adults at all stages of life learn how to prevent or reverse health issues through good nutrition, supplements, and a healthy lifestyle, showing how we can regain our vitality and blossom at any age.

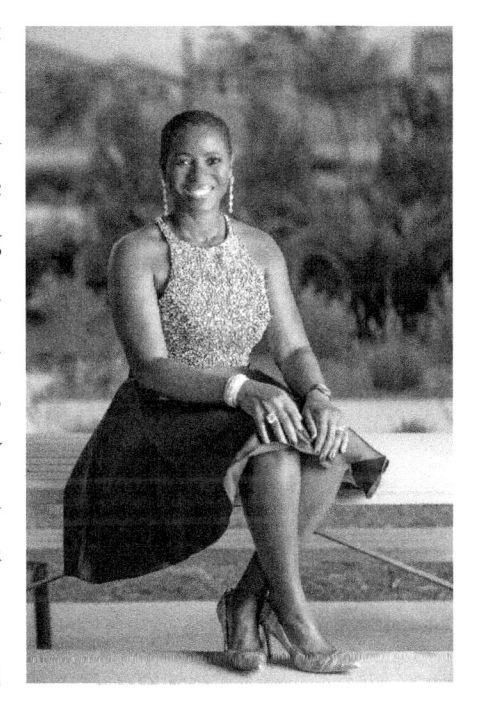

Sharing her own personal health challenges of being diagnosed with high blood pressure, only to be put on medication that delivered all sorts of side effects, she was determined to turn her life around through healthy eating and exercise. As an educator in universities, colleges, and elementary schools throughout the United States and Canada, she helps people realize how to rise above challenges and create a vision for a new life.

Nicoline says constant change is the only thing permanent in life; we do not have to remain stuck in our circumstances. We can think new thoughts, learn something new, and create healthy habits that make a difference in our lives.

Taking a firm initiative to use her challenging experiences to propel herself to a new level of growth, she learned that adversity can be our friend by providing us feedback for better performance in all areas of life. You, too, can make that new beginning by adopting the suggestions in this book. Welcome to your new life.

Printed in Great Britain
by Amazon